NCLEX: Oncology Nursing

105 Nursing Practice Questions & Rationales to
EASILY Crush the NCLEX!

Chase Hassen

Nurse Superhero

© 2015

Disclaimer:

Although the author and publisher have made every effort to ensure that the information in this book was correct at press time, the author and publisher do not assume and hereby disclaim any liability to any party for any loss, damage, or disruption caused by errors or omissions, whether such errors or omissions result from negligence, accident, or any other cause.

This book is not intended as a substitute for the medical advice of physicians. The reader should regularly consult a physician in matters relating to his/her health and particularly with respect to any symptoms that may require diagnosis or medical attention.

All rights reserved. No part of this publication may be reproduced, distributed, or transmitted in any form or by any means, including photocopying, recording, or other electronic or mechanical methods, without the prior written permission of the publisher, except in the case of brief quotations embodied in critical reviews and certain other noncommercial uses permitted by copyright law.

NCLEX®, NCLEX®-RN, and NCLEX®-PN are registered trademarks of the National Council of State Boards of Nursing, Inc. They hold no affiliation with this product.

© Copyright 2015 by Chase Hassen and Nurse Superhero. All rights reserved.

Have you seen my other NCLEX Prep Books?

NCLEX: Respiratory System : 105 Nursing Practice Questions and Rationales to Easily Crush the NCLEX!

NCLEX: Endocrine System : 105 Nursing Practice Questions and Rationales to EASILY Crush the NCLEX!

NCLEX: Cardiovascular System : 105 Nursing Practice and Rationales to Easily Crush the NCLEX!

NCLEX: Emergency Nursing : 105 Practice Questions and Rationales to Easily Crush the NCLEX!

EKG Interpretation: 24 Hours or Less to Easily Pass the ECG Portion of the NCLEX!

Lab Values: 137 Values You Know to Easily Pass The NCLEX!

First, I want to give you this FREE gift...

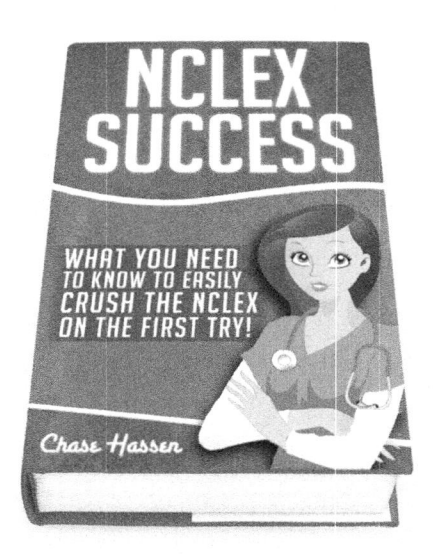

Just to say thanks for downloading my book, I wanted to give you another resource to help you absolutely crush the NCLEX Exam.

For a limited time you can download this book for FREE.

http://bit.ly/1VNGAZ9

Table of Contents

First, I want to give you this FREE gift... _____ 4
Chapter 1 : NCLEX: Oncology Questions _____ 6
Chapter 2 : NCLEX: Oncology Questions, Answers, and Rationales 60
Conclusion _____ 121
Highly Recommended Books for Success _____ 122

Oncology Nursing

Chapter 1 : NCLEX: Oncology Questions

The following are 105 questions that will help you study for the NCLEX evaluation. All of the questions are based on things you might need to know in the area of Oncology questions. Following the quiz will be the identical questions with the answers and rationales. Compare your answers with the correct ones to see where you may need to study some more. Good luck!

PLEASE NOTE: The answers are located in the next chapter. If you would prefer to see the questions and answers as you review this study guide, visit page 60.

1. The client has metastatic cancer and asks the nurse what it means to have metastatic cancer. What does the nurse say?
    a. Metastatic cancer involves having cancer spread through the blood or lymph vessels
    b. Metastatic cancer involves a reduction of blood vessels in the cancer.
    c. Metastatic cancer means that the cancer is fatal.
    d. Metastatic cancer is the easiest type of cancer to treat.

Answer:

2. The client has metastatic cancer and asks where the cancer has gone to. You tell the client that these are common areas of metastases. Select all that apply.
   a. Prostate gland
   b. Liver
   c. Brain
   d. Breast
   e. Lungs
   f. Bone

Answer:

3. The doctor has just told the client he has grade IV carcinoma. How do you explain grade IV carcinoma?
   a. Grade IV carcinoma represents cells that look much like normal cells.
   b. Grade IV carcinoma contains very immature and anaplastic cells.
   c. Grade IV carcinoma means that the cancer is fatal.
   d. Grade IV carcinoma means that the cells are moderately differentiated and slightly abnormal.

Answer:

4. The client has been told he has stage 0 cancer. How do you explain this stage of cancer to the client?
   a. Stage 0 cancer has very little chance of survival.
   b. Stage 0 cancer has lymph node involvement.
   c. Stage 0 cancer is always treated with chemotherapy alone.
   d. Stage 0 cancer is carcinoma in situ.

Answer:

5. The client has a T1N0M0 cancer. What does the nurse tell them about this type of cancer?
   a. The tumor is quite large and needs resection.
   b. The tumor has involvement of lymph nodes.
   c. The tumor has metastasized to another body area.
   d. The tumor is small, has no lymph node involvement and has not metastasized.

Answer:

6. The client wonders what the best way is to prevent colon cancer because it runs in his family. What do you say about preventing cancer?
   a. There is no way to prevent most cancers.
   b. Colon cancer is preventable through regular colonoscopies, starting at age 50.
   c. The best way to prevent colon cancer is educating the public about healthy eating
   d. Just eat a balanced diet of whole grains, fruits and vegetables and it will be okay.

Answer:

7. The client needs advice about doing a breast self-exam. What do you tell her? Select all that apply.
   a. Stand in front of the mirror with the hands and arms in different positions.
   b. Look for dimpling, prominent veins, puckered skin or flat nipples.
   c. There is no need to palpate the breast tissue.
   d. It does not help locate early breast cancers.
   e. Palpate the breast tissue in vertical or circular motions.
   f. Palpate the breast at least once a year for cancer.

Answer:

8. The client asks you about testicular self-examination. How do you educate the client? Select all that apply.
   a. The right testicle should weigh more than the left testicle.
   b. Roll each testicle between the first two fingers and the thumb.
   c. Perform while lying in bed.
   d. Men ages 20 and older should do this exam.
   e. The exam is looking for areas of increased veins in the testicles.
   f. The exam should be done in the shower with soapy hands.

Answer:

9. The client has been told to do a skin self-examination. What do you tell the client about skin self-exam?
   a. Everyone over the age of 60 should do this exam.
   b. You are looking for moles that haven't changed over the years.
   c. Skin tags are precancerous and you should talk to your doctor about getting them removed.
   d. You are systematically evaluating the skin for changes in the skin structures.

Answer:

Oncology Nursing

10. The client is scheduled for an incisional skin biopsy. You tell the client about the biopsy by saying:
    a. A needle will be used to obtain cells from the skin biopsy.
    b. The skin biopsy will remove less than the entire tumor.
    c. The tumor uses a punch to take out a section of skin.
    d. The tumor will be completely removed after the biopsy.

Answer:

11. The client is about to have a biopsy for cancer. What are some pre-procedure nursing interventions the nurse should do?
    a. All clients should be NPO.
    b. Give sedation if ordered and if the client is NPO.
    c. Make sure the client has someone to drive them home.
    d. Prepare the client to be hospitalized after the biopsy.

Answer:

12. The client is scheduled for imaging to identify the characteristics of the tumor. What does the nurse do to help the client prepare for the procedure?
   a. The client should be asked about allergies to contrast dye if this is to be used.
   b. Tell the client that the imaging should take no longer than 15 minutes.
   c. Tell the client that x-ray exposure is likely.
   d. Make sure the client is NPO.

Answer:

13. The client is having surgery for a possible tumor. What do you tell the client about the procedure?
   a. The procedure will be curative.
   b. The procedure will be used to biopsy the tissue.
   c. The surgery can be curative, palliative, diagnostic or used for staging.
   d. The client should have a person to drive them home after surgery.

Answer:

14. The client is scheduled to have radiation therapy for testicular cancer. What do you tell the client about this treatment?
    a. There will be pain medication available for the pain of radiation therapy.
    b. The testicular cells are particularly sensitive to radiation.
    c. Radiation kills cells through programmed cell death.
    d. The radiation will be done for palliative purposes.

Answer:

15. The client is scheduled for brachytherapy for his prostate cancer. What do you say to prepare the client for this type of therapy?
    a. An external beam of radiation will be directed at the prostate cells.
    b. The brachytherapy involves putting small seeds that are radioactive near the tumor.
    c. There will be markings on the skin to tell where the radiation should go.
    d. The client will have radiation 5 days a week for 4-6 weeks.

Answer:

16. The client should have what precautions taken when having brachytherapy?
    a. All bodily fluids should be considered radioactive.
    b. Pregnant nurses shouldn't care for clients undergoing brachytherapy.
    c. If an implant becomes dislodged, pick it up and replace it.
    d. Prepare for nausea, anorexia and fatigue.

Answer:

17. The client is having radiation to the lungs and wonders what the early symptoms might be. What do you tell them?
    a. The client may develop pulmonary fibrosis
    b. The client may develop a secondary malignancy.
    c. The client may have esophageal erosions.
    d. The client may have skin fibrosis.

Answer:

18. The client is scheduled for chemotherapy for testicular cancer. What do you tell the client about this procedure?
    a. It can be curative in testicular cancer.
    b. It is usually used in palliative situations.
    c. The chemotherapy is cell-cycle specific.
    d. The person's bodily fluids are considered hazardous.

Answer:

19. Biologic therapy for cancer is scheduled for the client. How do you explain biological therapy to the client?
    a. It is given intravenously.
    b. It can affect the immune system of the client.
    c. It is used to cure cancer.
    d. It is used instead of chemotherapy, radiation or surgery.

Answer:

20. The client is has AML and is scheduled to receive an allogenic bone marrow transplant. What do you tell the client about the allogenic transplant?
   a. The cells come from the client's own bone marrow stem cells.
   b. An umbilical cord blood sampling cannot be used.
   c. The donor must be an HLA match for the client.
   d. The client should not have chemotherapy before the transplant.

Answer:

21. The client is having an autologous transplant. How does the nurse explain this type of bone marrow transplant?
   a. The cells come from an HLA-matched donor.
   b. The cells come from stem cells harvested from the client.
   c. The client cannot receive chemotherapy before the procedure.
   d. The client cannot have radiation before the procedure.

Answer:

Oncology Nursing

22. You tell the client that there are complications of a stem cell transplant. What do you say?
    a. There can be host versus graft disease.
    b. There can be elevated levels of all cell types.
    c. There can be engrafting of the cells.
    d. There can be life-threatening bacterial, viral and fungal infections.

Answer:

23. You talk to the female client about the potential for having a child after total body irradiation. What do you say?
    a. There is a potential for second malignancy after the irradiation.
    b. The client will be sterile after the irradiation.
    c. The client under the age of 26 may still be fertile.
    d. The client should consider adoption.

Answer:

Oncology Nursing

24. The client is experiencing cancer pain. How does the nurse help the client? Select all that apply.
    a. Tell the client that narcotics are used as a last resort.
    b. Identify the intensity of the pain.
    c. Identify the specific source of the pain.
    d. Teach the client about narcotic use.
    e. Teach nonpharmacological methods of pain relief.
    f. Give the client narcotics whether or not they are experiencing pain.

Answer:

25. The client is experiencing a great deal of fatigue with cancer treatment. What does the nurse say or do?
    a. Tell the client that fatigue is uncommon in cancer treatment and will go away.
    b. Give the client a Piper Fatigue questionnaire
    c. Tell the client that rest will relieve the fatigue
    d. Give the client caffeine to counteract the fatigue

Answer:

Oncology Nursing

26. The client wants something to improve the fatigue of chemotherapy. What can the nurse give?
    a. Erythropoietin
    b. Caffeine
    c. Phenobarbital
    d. Tell them there is no treatment for the fatigue.

Answer:

27. The client has neutropenia as a result of chemotherapy. You recognize that neutropenia involves a WBC count of less than what value?
    a. 4000
    b. 3000
    c. 2000
    d. 1000

Answer:

28. The nurse is monitoring the client for signs of infection after chemotherapy. The most reliable indicator of infection is what?
   a. Neutrophilia
   b. Fever of a degree or more above normal
   c. Mental status changes
   d. Bruising

Answer:

29. The family of a chemotherapy client asks about prevention of infection. What does the nurse say?
   a. The family should take antibiotics to prevent spread of infection.
   b. The client and family should practice strict handwashing techniques
   c. The family should wear a gown, gloves and mask when dealing with the client
   d. Children are not allowed to see the client.

Answer:

Oncology Nursing

30. The client has a fever and chills after chemotherapy. What does the nurse give? Select all that apply.
    a. Aspirin
    b. Acetaminophen
    c. Demerol
    d. Erythropoietin
    e. Ibuprofen
    f. Naproxen

Answer:

31. The client is having nausea from chemotherapy. What nursing interventions do you do?
    a. Tell the client to take antiemetics when vomiting.
    b. Instruct the client on relaxation techniques.
    c. Tell the client to lie down after eating.
    d. Tell the client to eat more sweet and spicy foods.

Answer:

32. The client has stomatitis after chemotherapy. What can you tell the client?
   a. Use viscous xylocaine for pain relief.
   b. Eat plenty of popcorn and nuts.
   c. Suck on hard candy.
   d. Chew gum.

Answer:

33. The client is having constipation after chemotherapy. As the nurse, what do you suggest?
   a. Avoid taking in fiber
   b. Avoid dairy products
   c. Take in extra dietary fiber
   d. Restrict fluids

Answer:

34. The client is having problems coping because of her cancer diagnosis. How can the nurse help? Select all that apply.
    a. Assess for suicide plans.
    b. Assess for homicide plans.
    c. Get a psychiatric and substance abuse history.
    d. Encourage alcohol use in order to cope.
    e. Monitor the client for evidence of depression.
    f. Tell the client the symptoms will pass without intervention.

Answer:

35. A client is suffering from electrolyte complications of cancer. What is the most common electrolyte complication of cancer?
    a. Hypokalemia
    b. Hypocalcemia
    c. Hypernatremia
    d. Hypercalcemia

Answer:

36. The client is suffering from hypercalcemia from cancer. What does the nurse do about medications?
    a. Give bisphosphonates.
    b. Give extra digoxin.
    c. Avoid narcotic pain relief.
    d. Give medications with milk.

Answer:

37. The client with cancer has had mediastinal lymphadenopathy and has developed a sudden onset of shortness of breath, head swelling, swelling of the eyes, severe headache, neck, and arm swelling. What is most likely going on?
    a. Pulmonary embolism
    b. Pneumothorax
    c. Superior vena cava syndrome
    d. Rupture of the abdominal aorta

Answer:

Oncology Nursing

38. The client has small cell cancer of the lung and has had a weight gain of greater than 5 pounds in one day, nausea and vomiting, confusion, fatigue, a serum sodium of 125 and decreased urinary output. What might be going on?
    a. Small cell cancer making inappropriate amounts of antidiuretic hormone (SIADH)
    b. Has been given too much IV fluids
    c. Kidney failure
    d. Kidney involvement in cancer

Answer:

39. The client has SIADH from cancer. What are some nursing interventions that might be done?
    a. Increase IV fluids.
    b. Monitor blood for electrolyte imbalance.
    c. Give sugarless candy to better handle fluid restriction.
    d. Give hypotonic saline to bring down sodium level.
    e. Obtain daily weights.
    f. Give the client a high salt diet.

Answer:

40. A client with leukemia has the acute onset of muscle twitching, seizures, lethargy, confusion and cardiac arrhythmias after receiving chemotherapy. What is going on?
    a. The client is having hypercalcemia from cancer.
    b. The client is suffering from tumor lysis syndrome.
    c. The client is getting too little fluid.
    d. The client is suffering from hypokalemia.

Answer:

41. The smoking client has gross hematuria that is painless and suprapubic, rectal and back pain. What do you suspect?
    a. Prostatitis
    b. UTI
    c. Transitional cell cancer of the bladder
    d. Pyelonephritis

Answer:

Oncology Nursing

42. The client has superficial transitional cell cancer of the bladder. What treatment would he likely get?
    a. Transurethral resection of the tumor and destruction of surrounding tumor.
    b. Radical cystectomy with removal of bladder, prostate, urethra, and seminal vesicles
    c. Brachytherapy
    d. BCG given intravesically for six weeks

Answer:

43. The male client is a smoker and has had excessive occupational exposure to lead cadmium and hematuria. What kind of cancer is he likely to have?
    a. Renal cell cancer
    b. Prostate cancer
    c. Bladder cancer
    d. Urethral cancer

Answer:

Oncology Nursing

44. The client has metastatic renal cell cancer. What can you tell the client about sites of metastases?
    a. It usually spreads to the brain.
    b. It spreads by direct extension to the renal vein or vena cava.
    c. It usually spreads to the other kidney.
    d. It usually spreads via the blood to the bladder.

Answer:

45. The female client has been diagnosed with breast cancer. What do you tell the client in order to educate her?
    a. It is the third most common cancer in women.
    b. Most cancers occur in the inner lower quadrant.
    c. Stage I and stage II disease are 70-90 percent curable.
    d. It is not capable of metastasis.

Answer:

46. The 75 year old female client has a red breast, with an orange-peel appearance to the skin and a painful breast. What could be going on?
   a. Ductal breast cancer
   b. Inflammatory breast cancer
   c. Lobular breast cancer
   d. Mastitis

Answer:

47. The client wants to know the most common areas of metastasis for her breast cancer? What do you say?
   a. Bone marrow, kidney, adrenal glands, gallbladder
   b. Bone, lung, liver, brain
   c. Brain only
   d. Intestines, pancreas, the other breast, gallbladder

Answer:

48. The client tells you she is scheduled for a simple mastectomy for her breast cancer and asks you what this means. What do you tell her?
   a. It involves the removal of the lump and some surrounding breast tissue.
   b. It involves the removal of the entire breast, including the nipple and the skin.
   c. It involves removal of the breast, the nipple, the skin and the axillary lymph nodes.
   d. It involves removal of the breast tissue, skin, lymph nodes and pectoral muscles.

Answer:

49. The client with breast cancer is to have a sentinel lymph node biopsy. What do you tell her about this procedure?
   a. The largest lymph node in the axilla is removed to look for cancer.
   b. All the lymph nodes of the axilla are removed to look for cancer.
   c. Dye is injected in the lymph system, looking for the first draining axillary lymph node.
   d. Any lymph nodes that look suspicious for cancer are removed from the axilla.

Answer:

50. The client is scheduled for radiation following lumpectomy. How do you educate the client abut this procedure?
   a. Tiny beads of radioactivity will be put beneath the skin at the time of surgery.
   b. Radiation is done during surgery to remove the breast.
   c. Radiation is done six months after the lump is removed if there is evidence of the cancer returning.
   d. External beam radiation is done about three weeks after the lump is removed.

Answer:

51. The patient is being given Herceptin after treatment of breast cancer. How does the nurse explain the role of Herceptin?
   a. Tell her it is a form of chemotherapy for breast cancer.
   b. Tell her it is used to get rid of any cancer cells that weren't removed in surgery.
   c. Tell her it is a monoclonal antibody therapy used for tumors that express the HER2 oncogene.
   d. Tell her it is a hormone that blocks the growth of breast cancer cells.

Answer:

52. The client recently underwent a CT scan for headaches that showed a mass on the brain. What do you tell the client about the brain mass?
    a. It is likely to be a malignant tumor.
    b. It is almost always fatal.
    c. Surgery will be used to remove the tumor.
    d. There are more metastatic brain cancers than primary brain cancers.

Answer:

53. The client has a metastatic brain tumor. He asks about the most common way of treating this type of condition. How do you respond?
    a. Most metastatic brain tumors are treated with radiation therapy.
    b. Most metastatic brain tumors are treated with chemotherapy.
    c. Most metastatic brain tumors are treated with stereotactic surgery.
    d. Most metastatic brain tumors are not treated at all.

Answer:

Oncology Nursing

54. The client with cervical cancer asks about her risk factors for the disease. What do you tell her about her risk factors? Select all that apply.
    a. Cigarette smoking is a risk factor.
    b. Human papillomavirus is a risk factor.
    c. Alcohol intake is a risk factor.
    d. High socioeconomic status is a risk factor
    e. Having multiple sex partners is a risk factor.
    f. Having sex after age 21 is a risk factor.

Answer:

55. The client is wondering about the best way to avoid getting cervical cancer. What do you say on prevention of cervical cancer?
    a. Avoid alcohol intake.
    b. Get a Pap smear upon becoming sexually active.
    c. Avoid douches.
    d. Get a routine colposcopy every 5 years.

Answer:

56. The client is scheduled for a colposcopy. What do you tell the client in the way of education about colposcopy?
    a. Colposcopy is done under general anesthesia.
    b. Colposcopy involves putting a tube up the vagina and visualizing the cervix.
    c. Colposcopy involves putting acetic acid on the cervix and visualizing it under magnification.
    d. Colposcopy always results in removal of the cervix at the time of the procedure.

Answer:

57. A 55 year old woman is diagnosed with cervical cancer. What is the main treatment of choice?
    a. Radiation to the pelvis.
    b. Removal of the cervix with sparing of the uterus.
    c. Cone biopsy of the cervix.
    d. Total abdominal hysterectomy and lymphadenectomy.

Answer:

58. Nursing interventions for a client treated for cervical cancer include the following. Select all that apply?
    a. Measure all intake and output.
    b. Bladder retraining using a suprapubic catheter.
    c. Douche every 24 hours
    d. Assess for changes in bowel and bladder pattern after surgery/radiation.
    e. Avoid sex for 6 weeks.
    f. Teach how to use tampons after surgery.

Answer:

59. The client has been diagnosed with colon cancer and asks why he got the disease. What do you say in terms of risk factors for colon cancer?
    a. Eating a diet high in fish is a risk factor.
    b. Having a positive family history is a risk factor.
    c. Lupus is a risk factor.
    d. Eating lots of vegetables is a risk factor.

Answer:

60. The client has metastatic colon cancer. What is the most common site of metastatic colon cancer?
   a. Brain
   b. Pancreas
   c. Liver
   d. Lung

Answer:

61. The client is asked about the best prevention of colon cancer. What do you tell the client?
   a. Drink no more than 2 alcoholic beverages per day.
   b. Have a FIT test every five years.
   c. Be seen if there is blood from the rectum.
   d. Have a colonoscopy every ten years after age 50.

Answer:

Oncology Nursing

62. The client is having surgery to remove colon cancer the next day. What does the nurse expect to do?
   a. Give a Dulcolax suppository the night before the surgery.
   b. Give a GoLytely prep the day before the surgery.
   c. Give IV antibiotics on the day before the procedure.
   d. Restrict fluids the day before the procedure.

Answer:

63. The client has colon cancer in the sigmoid colon. What procedure is the client likely to have to treat this condition?
   a. Left hemicolectomy
   b. Sigmoidectomy
   c. Right hemicolectomy
   d. Total colectomy

Answer:

64. Priority nursing interventions for a client who is undergoing colon surgery for colon cancer includes:
    a. Tell them to expect normal sexual function after recovery.
    b. Watch for an anastomotic leak from the site of the surgical re-connect.
    c. Educate the client on eating after surgery.
    d. Monitor for bladder dysfunction.

Answer:

65. The client is at risk for endometrial cancer. What are her risks?
    a. Being younger than age 30.
    b. Having multiple children.
    c. Being African-American.
    d. Having a family history of breast or ovarian cancer.

Answer:

66. Common metastatic sites for endometrial cancer include the following:
    a. Cervix and vagina
    b. Colon
    c. Liver
    d. Brain

Answer:

67. The best method of detecting endometrial cancer is what?
    a. A Pap smear
    b. An endometrial biopsy
    c. A hysterectomy
    d. Vaginal washings

Answer:

68. The client has gastric cancer and wonders about his risks for getting the disease. What are they?
   a. Female gender
   b. Being Caucasian
   c. Having a Helicobacter infection
   d. Having colon cancer

Answer:

69. The client has metastatic gastric cancer. Where is a likely metastasis?
   a. Pancreas
   b. Bone
   c. Brain
   d. Lung

Answer:

Oncology Nursing

70. The client has cancer of the larynx and wonders how he got it. What is a main risk factor for laryngeal cancer?
    a. Eating a low fiber diet
    b. Having laryngeal polyps
    c. Smoking history
    d. Illicit drug use

Answer:

71. The client has metastatic cancer of the larynx. Where is the major site of metastasis?
    a. Bone
    b. Brain
    c. Other head and neck areas
    d. Colon

Answer:

72. The client has persistent hoarseness, throat pain, and a painless mass in the neck. What is the most likely diagnosis?
    a. Laryngeal polyp
    b. Laryngeal cancer
    c. Tonsillitis
    d. Esophagitis

Answer:

73. The client has nasopharyngeal cancer. What can he expect as the main form of therapy?
    a. Removal of the voice box.
    b. Radiation to the head and neck.
    c. Interleukin-2
    d. Cisplatin

Answer:

Oncology Nursing

74. The client has weight loss, unexplained bleeding, splenomegaly, anemia, low platelet count and a WBC count of 50,000. What do you expect is going on?
    a. Hodgkin's lymphoma
    b. Anorexia nervosa
    c. Non-Hodgkin's lymphoma
    d. Acute leukemia

Answer:

75. The primary treatment for leukemia and multiple myeloma is what?
    a. Lymph node surgery
    b. Chemotherapy alone
    c. Chemotherapy and radiation
    d. Chemotherapy and bone marrow transplant

Answer:

76. The client has been diagnosed with lung cancer and wonders how he got it. What does the nurse say about the primary cause of lung cancer?
    a. Cigarette smoking
    b. Radon gas
    c. Asbestos exposure
    d. Secondhand smoke

Answer:

77. The client is suspected of having lung cancer by a suspicious x-ray of the chest. What follow up test is most appropriate to detect whether or not the suspicious area is cancer?
    a. Repeat CXR in six months.
    b. Bronchoscopy with biopsy.
    c. Sputum culture.
    d. Lobectomy of the lung.

Answer:

78. The client has been diagnosed with localized small cell cancer. What is the standard treatment for this disease?
   a. Pneumonectomy
   b. Lobectomy
   c. Chemotherapy
   d. Brachytherapy

Answer:

79. Nursing interventions for those who have had a lobectomy for lung cancer include the following:
   a. Lie on the side of the operation for better drainage.
   b. Encourage a reduction in smoking.
   c. Manage chest tubes in lobectomy.
   d. Keep the client in bed for at least a week.

Answer:

80. The client has been diagnosed with ovarian cancer. How do you educate the client about the disease?
    a. The peak age is 80-89 years of age.
    b. A total of 60-70 percent of people are diagnosed at stage III or IV.
    c. Being multiparous is a risk factor.
    d. The five year survival rate is 80 percent.

Answer:

81. The client has metastatic cervical cancer. Where are the most likely site(s) for metastasis of this type of cancer?
    a. Extension to fallopian tubes, uterus, bladder and peritoneum
    b. Bone
    c. Brain
    d. Liver

Answer:

82. The routine treatment for ovarian cancer is what?
    a. Brachytherapy at the site of cancer
    b. Radiation to the abdomen
    c. Total abdominal hysterectomy and bilateral oophorectomy
    d. Chemotherapy in the peritoneum

Answer:

83. The client has discovered he has prostate cancer and wants to know details. How do you educate him on the disease?
    a. It has the highest rate in Caucasians.
    b. It has a nearly 100 percent 5 year survival rate.
    c. It is the leading cause of cancer death in men.
    d. It is most common in men under the age of 65.

Answer:

84. The client has metastatic prostate cancer. What is the major site of prostate cancer metastases?
    a. Bone
    b. Brain
    c. Pancreas
    d. Omentum

Answer:

85. The client has a weak urinary stream and an inability to start or stop the flow of urine. He has frequent nocturia and hematuria. What kind of cancer might he have?
    a. Bladder cancer
    b. Kidney cancer
    c. Urethral cancer
    d. Prostate cancer

Answer:

86. Surgical management of prostate cancer include what?
    a. Radical prostatectomy
    b. Lymph node removal of the pelvic lymph nodes
    c. Transurethral resection of the prostate
    d. Only radiation surgery is recommended

Answer:

87. Adjuvant therapy for prostate cancer includes:
    a. Removal of urethra.
    b. External beam radiation of the bladder
    c. Hormonal manipulation
    d. Removal of the bladder

Answer:

88. Nursing interventions for prostate cancer clients include the following:
   a. Teach the client how to remove the catheter after surgery.
   b. Keep client in bed for 48 hours after surgery.
   c. Give laxatives for constipation.
   d. Report to physician if client has evidence of infection after brachytherapy.

Answer:

89. After brachytherapy for prostate cancer, the client should be instructed by telling him this:
   a. The brachytherapy seeds pose a hazard to those around him.
   b. The client can be around pregnant women after receiving brachytherapy.
   c. Strain the urine for dislodged seeds.
   d. The client can be discharged immediately after receiving brachytherapy.

Answer:

Oncology Nursing

90. The client has been diagnosed with skin cancer. How do you educate the client as to skin cancer?
    a. Melanoma is the most common type of skin cancer.
    b. Basal cell carcinoma is often fatal.
    c. Seborrheic keratoses can lead to squamous cell cancer.
    d. Actinic keratoses can lead to squamous cell cancer.

Answer:

91. The client has been diagnosed with melanoma. How do you educate the client on melanoma?
    a. The rate is highest among African-Americans.
    b. The melanoma arises from cells in the epidermis.
    c. It is more common in women than men.
    d. It cannot be prevented.

Answer:

92. Risk factors for melanoma include:
    a. Wearing sunscreen in adulthood only.
    b. Getting bad sunburns in childhood.
    c. Having a darker complexion
    d. Getting sunburn in older age.

Answer:

93. Melanoma can be identified by what characteristics?
    a. Non-uniform color of lesions
    b. Symmetric expansion of a mole
    c. Regular borders in the mole.
    d. Pearly appearance to the nodule.

Answer:

94. Treatment of a basal cell or squamous cell skin cancer includes:
    a. Radiation only
    b. Punch biopsy to the lesion.
    c. Wide excision to include healthy tissue
    d. Chemotherapy only

Answer:

95. Common adjuvant therapy for melanoma cancer includes:
    a. External beam radiation
    b. Brachytherapy
    c. Chemotherapy
    d. Removal of lymph nodes

Answer:

Oncology Nursing

96. The patient has been diagnosed with osteosarcoma. Where is the tumor originating from?
    a. Cartilage
    b. Bone
    c. Fibrous tissue
    d. Reticuloendothelial tissue

Answer:

97. The client has been diagnosed with osteosarcoma. How do you educate the client with regard to this tumor?
    a. It is a common form of cancer.
    b. It is the most common bone tumor.
    c. The survival rate is 25 percent after five years.
    d. It does not require chemotherapy.

Answer:

98. The client has osteosarcoma and wonders about risk factors for the disease. What do you say?
    a. It is most common after the age of 50.
    b. It is most common in females.
    c. Previous radiation is a risk factor.
    d. Older adults never get the disease.

Answer:

99. The client has metastatic osteosarcoma. What do you say about the most common metastatic sites?
    a. It is mostly metastatic to lungs.
    b. It is most metastatic to brain.
    c. It is most metastatic to liver.
    d. It is most metastatic to bowel tissue.

Answer:

Oncology Nursing

100. Nursing interventions for soft tissue sarcomas include what? Select all that apply.
   a. Emotional support for changes in body image.
   b. Increase fluids after surgery.
   c. Collaborate with speech therapy.
   d. Teach transfer techniques after surgery.
   e. Prepare the client for phantom limb pain if amputation is done.
   f. Monitor electrolytes.

Answer:

101. The client has been diagnosed with testicular cancer. How do you educate the client about this type of cancer?
   a. It is a common male cancer.
   b. It occurs most often in men between the ages of 15 and 35.
   c. It is a non-aggressive tumor.
   d. It has the highest incidence in African-Americans.

Answer:

102. The male client has found a small, hard scrotal mass. What do you suspect?
   a. Varicocele
   b. Testicular cancer
   c. Undescended testicle
   d. Testicular torsion

Answer:

103. A common blood test for testicular cancer is what?
   a. Serum alkaline phosphatase
   b. Serum CA-125
   c. Serum LDH level
   d. Serum beta HCG

Answer:

104. The client asks the nurse about mortality from cancer. How does the nurse respond?
   a. About 5 million people in the US survive cancer for five years or more.
   b. Everyone in the US with cancer will eventually die from their disease.
   c. Cancer is the leading cause of adult death in the US.
   d. Do not discuss mortality with clients who have cancer.

Answer:

105. The client indicates that he has heard that all men get prostate cancer at some point in their lives. How does the nurse educate the client?
   a. Lung cancer is the most frequently diagnosed cancer in men.
   b. Prostate cancer is the most frequently diagnosed cancer in men.
   c. Prostate cancer is most common in Caucasian men.
   d. As there is no way to screen for prostate cancer, it is the number one cause of cancer death in men.

Answer:

Great Job! On the next chapter, you will see the questions you just answered plus the answers and rationales! I hope you did well!

Chapter 2 : NCLEX: Oncology Questions, Answers, and Rationales

The following are the same questions you just took with the answers and rationales. Compare your answers with the correct answers to see where you may need to study further.

1. The client has metastatic cancer and asks the nurse what it means to have metastatic cancer. What does the nurse say?
   a. Metastatic cancer involves having cancer spread through the blood or lymph vessels
   b. Metastatic cancer involves a reduction of blood vessels in the cancer.
   c. Metastatic cancer means that the cancer is fatal.
   d. Metastatic cancer is the easiest type of cancer to treat.

Answer: a. Metastatic cancer involves growth and development of blood vessels along with spread of the cancer through blood or lymph vessels to reach other body areas. It is not uniformly fatal and it is usually more difficult to treat than localized cancer.

2. The client has metastatic cancer and asks where the cancer has gone to. You tell the client that these are the four most common areas of metastases. Select all that apply.
   a. Prostate gland
   b. Liver
   c. Brain
   d. Breast
   e. Lungs
   f. Bone

Answer: b. c. e. f. The liver, brain, lungs and bone are the most common sites for metastases.

3. The doctor has just told the client he has grade IV carcinoma. How do you explain grade IV carcinoma?
   a. Grade IV carcinoma represents cells that look much like normal cells.
   b. Grade IV carcinoma contains very immature and anaplastic cells.
   c. Grade IV carcinoma means that the cancer is fatal.
   d. Grade IV carcinoma means that the cells are moderately differentiated and slightly abnormal.

Answer: b. In grade IV carcinoma, the cells are very immature and anaplastic so that it is difficult to identify the origin of the cancer. It is not always fatal. Grade I carcinoma has cells that look much like normal cells and grade II carcinoma contains moderately differentiated and slightly abnormal cells.

4. The client has been told he has stage 0 cancer. How do you explain this stage of cancer to the client?
   a. Stage 0 cancer has very little chance of survival.
   b. Stage 0 cancer has lymph node involvement.
   c. Stage 0 cancer is always treated with chemotherapy alone.
   d. Stage 0 cancer is carcinoma in situ.

Answer: d. Stage 0 cancer is carcinoma in situ. It has a good chance of survival and doesn't involve the lymph nodes. Stage 0 cancer can be treated in different ways, including surgery, radiation, or chemotherapy.

Oncology Nursing

5. The client has a T1N0M0 cancer. What does the nurse tell them about this type of cancer?
   a. The tumor is quite large and needs resection.
   b. The tumor has involvement of lymph nodes.
   c. The tumor has metastasized to another body area.
   d. The tumor is small, has no lymph node involvement and has not metastasized.

Answer: d. The T1N0M0 cancer is small in size (T1), has no lymph node involvement (N0), and no metastases (M0). This is a tumor classification system used to identify the characteristics of a cancer.

6. The client wonders what the best way is to prevent colon cancer because it runs in his family. What do you say about preventing cancer?
   a. There is no way to prevent most cancers.
   b. Colon cancer is preventable through regular colonoscopies, starting at age 50.
   c. The best way to prevent colon cancer is educating the public about healthy eating
   d. Just eat a balanced diet of whole grains, fruits and vegetables and it will be okay.

Answer: b. Colon cancer is preventable through getting regular colonoscopies, starting at age 50, sooner if there is a family history. Many cancers can be prevented through screening. Eating a healthy diet does help in the prevention of some cancers.

7. The client needs advice about doing a breast self-exam. What do you tell her? Select all that apply.
   a. Stand in front of the mirror with the hands and arms in different positions.
   b. Look for dimpling, prominent veins, puckered skin or flat nipples.
   c. There is no need to palpate the breast tissue.
   d. It does not help locate early breast cancers.
   e. Palpate the breast tissue in vertical or circular motions.
   f. Palpate the breast at least once a year for cancer.

Answer: a. b. e. A breast self-exam is a monthly exam used to detect early cancers. The woman stands in front of a mirror or is lying down with the arms and hands in different positions. The breast is observed for dimpling, puckering, prominent veins or flat nipples. The palpation can be circular or vertical.

Oncology Nursing

8. The client asks you about testicular self-examination. How do you educate the client? Select all that apply.
   a. The right testicle should weigh more than the left testicle.
   b. Roll each testicle between the first two fingers and the thumb.
   c. Perform while lying in bed.
   d. Men ages 20 and older should do this exam.
   e. The exam is looking for areas of increased veins in the testicles.
   f. The exam should be done in the shower with soapy hands.

Answer: b. f. Men over the age of 40 should do this exam and should check for nodules in the testicles by comparing the weight of the two testicles (which should be equal) and by rolling the testicle between the first two fingers and the thumb.

9. The client has been told to do a skin self-examination. What do you tell the client about skin self-exam?
   a. Everyone over the age of 60 should do this exam.
   b. You are looking for moles that haven't changed over the years.
   c. Skin tags are precancerous and you should talk to your doctor about getting them removed.
   d. You are systematically evaluating the skin for changes in the skin structures.

Answer: d. The exam should be done in anyone over the age of 30. You are systematically evaluating the skin for changes in the skin structures. Moles that haven't changed are not considered dangerous nor are skin tags.

Oncology Nursing

10. The client is scheduled for an incisional skin biopsy. You tell the client about the biopsy by saying:
    a. A needle will be used to obtain cells from the skin biopsy.
    b. The skin biopsy will remove less than the entire tumor.
    c. The tumor uses a punch to take out a section of skin.
    d. The tumor will be completely removed after the biopsy.

Answer: b. In an incisional biopsy, less than the entire tumor is taken. A punch biopsy uses a punch device to get a core out of the suspicious tissue. The tumor is removed entirely, only with an excisional biopsy.

Oncology Nursing

11. The client is about to have a biopsy for cancer. What are some pre-procedure nursing interventions the nurse should do?
    a. All clients should be NPO.
    b. Give sedation if ordered and if the client is NPO.
    c. Make sure the client has someone to drive them home.
    d. Prepare the client to be hospitalized after the biopsy.

Answer: b. If the client is NPO, which is not always necessary, sedation may be ordered. The client only needs to be driven home if they have been sedated. Hospitalization is not always necessary after a biopsy.

12. The client is scheduled for imaging to identify the characteristics of the tumor. What does the nurse do to help the client prepare for the procedure?
    a. The client should be asked about allergies to contrast dye if this is to be used.
    b. Tell the client that the imaging should take no longer than 15 minutes.
    c. Tell the client that x-ray exposure is likely.
    d. Make sure the client is NPO.

Answer: a. If dye is used, the client should be asked about allergies to contrast dye. The procedure can take between 30-120 minutes. The client may or may not have x-ray exposure and being NPO is a part of only some imaging procedures.

Oncology Nursing

13. The client is having surgery for a possible tumor. What do you tell the client about the procedure?
    a. The procedure will be curative.
    b. The procedure will be used to biopsy the tissue.
    c. The surgery can be curative, palliative, diagnostic or used for staging.
    d. The client should have a person to drive them home after surgery.

Answer: c. The surgery can be curative, palliative, diagnostic or for staging. The client may be hospitalized so it may not be a same day procedure. Not all surgeries are for biopsy or curing the patient.

14. The client is scheduled to have radiation therapy for testicular cancer. What do you tell the client about this treatment?
    a. There will be pain medication available for the pain of radiation therapy.
    b. The testicular cells are particularly sensitive to radiation.
    c. Radiation kills cells through programmed cell death.
    d. The radiation will be done for palliative purposes.

Answer: b. Testicular cells are particularly sensitive to radiation. The radiation generally doesn't hurt and it kills by disrupting mitosis. Radiation may not be done for palliative purposes.

Oncology Nursing

15. The client is scheduled for brachytherapy for his prostate cancer. What do you say to prepare the client for this type of therapy?
    a. An external beam of radiation will be directed at the prostate cells.
    b. The brachytherapy involves putting small seeds that are radioactive near the tumor.
    c. There will be markings on the skin to tell where the radiation should go.
    d. The client will have radiation 5 days a week for 4-6 weeks.

Answer: b. Brachytherapy involves putting radioactive seeds near the prostate cancer. They are simply placed there and left in so frequent visits to the radiation center are not necessary. Markings on the skin are not necessary.

16. The client should have what precautions taken when having brachytherapy?
    a. All bodily fluids should be considered radioactive.
    b. Pregnant nurses shouldn't care for clients undergoing brachytherapy.
    c. If an implant becomes dislodged, pick it up and replace it.
    d. Prepare for nausea, anorexia and fatigue.

Answer: b. Pregnant nurses shouldn't care for clients undergoing brachytherapy. Bodily fluids are not radioactive if the person is undergoing brachytherapy. If an implant becomes dislodged, pick it up with a long forceps and store it in a radioactive-proof container. There are not usually systemic signs with brachytherapy.

17. The client is having radiation to the lungs and wonders what the early symptoms might be. What do you tell them?
    a. The client may develop pulmonary fibrosis
    b. The client may develop a secondary malignancy.
    c. The client may have esophageal erosions.
    d. The client may have skin fibrosis.

Answer: c. An early symptom of radiation treatment includes esophageal erosions, especially when the lungs are treated. Late findings (past 6 months) include pulmonary fibrosis, a secondary malignancy, and skin fibrosis.

Oncology Nursing

18. The client is scheduled for chemotherapy for testicular cancer. What do you tell the client about this procedure?
    a. It can be curative in testicular cancer.
    b. It is usually used in palliative situations.
    c. The chemotherapy is cell-cycle specific.
    d. The person's bodily fluids are considered hazardous.

Answer: a. Chemotherapy can be curative in testicular cancer. It is not always palliative and the chemotherapy can be cell-cycle specific or cell-cycle nonspecific. The person's bodily fluids are not considered hazardous if disposed of properly.

19. Biologic therapy for cancer is scheduled for the client. How do you explain biological therapy to the client?
    a. It is given intravenously.
    b. It can affect the immune system of the client.
    c. It is used to cure cancer.
    d. It is used instead of chemotherapy, radiation or surgery.

Answer: b. Biologic therapy can affect the immune system of the client or can kill cancer cells directly. It can be given by several routes, including oral routes. It can be used to cure, control, or maintain the cancer. It can be used along with chemotherapy, radiation, and cancer.

20. The client is has AML and is scheduled to receive an allogenic bone marrow transplant. What do you tell the client about the allogenic transplant?
   a. The cells come from the client's own bone marrow stem cells.
   b. An umbilical cord blood sampling cannot be used.
   c. The donor must be an HLA match for the client.
   d. The client should not have chemotherapy before the transplant.

Answer: c. In an allogenic bone marrow transplant, the client's relatives or an unrelated donor match can be used as long as the HLA type matches the client. Umbilical cord blood can be enough but may not have enough volume. The client usually has high dose chemotherapy before the transplant.

21. The client is having an autologous transplant. How does the nurse explain this type of bone marrow transplant?
    a. The cells come from an HLA-matched donor.
    b. The cells come from stem cells harvested from the client.
    c. The client cannot receive chemotherapy before the procedure.
    d. The client cannot have radiation before the procedure.

Answer: b. The cells come from stem cells that come from the client and have been purged of tumor cells. It is often used in treating leukemia, lymphomas, and several types of solid tumors. Chemotherapy and sometimes radiation are used prior to giving back the stem cells.

22. You tell the client that there are complications of a stem cell transplant. What do you say?
    a. There can be host versus graft disease.
    b. There can be elevated levels of all cell types.
    c. There can be engrafting of the cells.
    d. There can be life-threatening bacterial, viral and fungal infections.

Answer: d. Complications of a stem cell transplant include graft versus host disease, failure to engraft the cells, or a life-threatening bacterial, viral, and fungal infections.

23. You talk to the female client about the potential for having a child after total body irradiation. What do you say?
   a. There is a potential for second malignancy after the irradiation.
   b. The client will be sterile after the irradiation.
   c. The client under the age of 26 may still be fertile.
   d. The client should consider adoption.

Answer: c. With regard to the potential to have a child, you can tell the client that if she is under the age of 26, she may still be fertile. There is a chance for a secondary malignancy but this does not apply to sterility.

24. The client is experiencing cancer pain. How does the nurse help the client? Select all that apply.
   a. Tell the client that narcotics are used as a last resort.
   b. Identify the intensity of the pain.
   c. Identify the specific source of the pain.
   d. Teach the client about narcotic use.
   e. Teach nonpharmacological methods of pain relief.
   f. Give the client narcotics whether or not they are experiencing pain.

Answer: b. d. e. The nurse should identify the intensity of the pain but the specific source is not necessary. Narcotics do not need to be used as a last resort but are not needed if there is no pain. Nonpharmacological methods of pain relief should be taught.

Oncology Nursing

25. The client is experiencing a great deal of fatigue with cancer treatment. What does the nurse say or do?
    a. Tell the client that fatigue is uncommon in cancer treatment and will go away.
    b. Give the client a Piper Fatigue questionnaire
    c. Tell the client that rest will relieve the fatigue
    d. Give the client caffeine to counteract the fatigue

Answer: b. The nurse can give the client a Piper Fatigue questionnaire. Fatigue is the most common symptom of cancer treatment. Rest and caffeine do not counteract or relieve the pain.

26. The client wants something to improve the fatigue of chemotherapy. What can the nurse give?
    a. Erythropoietin
    b. Caffeine
    c. Phenobarbital
    d. Tell them there is no treatment for the fatigue.

Answer: a. Good treatments for the fatigue of chemotherapy are erythropoietin, oxygen, and blood products to help anemia and oxygenation. Caffeine and phenobarbital will not help relieve the fatigue.

27. The client has neutropenia as a result of chemotherapy. You recognize that neutropenia involves a WBC count of less than what value?
   a. 4000
   b. 3000
   c. 2000
   d. 1000

Answer: d. Absolute neutropenia involves a WBC count of less than 1000/ml.

28. The nurse is monitoring the client for signs of infection after chemotherapy. The most reliable indicator of infection is what?
   a. Neutrophilia
   b. Fever of a degree or more above normal
   c. Mental status changes
   d. Bruising

Answer: b. The most reliable indicator of infection is a fever of a degree or more above normal. The neutrophil count is generally low after chemotherapy. Mental status changes can be from other sources and bruising is a sign of thrombocytopenia after chemotherapy.

Oncology Nursing

29. The family of a chemotherapy client asks about prevention of infection. What does the nurse say?
    a. The family should take antibiotics to prevent spread of infection.
    b. The client and family should practice strict handwashing techniques
    c. The family should wear a gown, gloves and mask when dealing with the client
    d. Children are not allowed to see the client.

Answer: b. The client and family should practice strict handwashing techniques. A gown, gloves, and mask are usually not required. The family does not need to take antibiotics and children who are not ill may see the client.

30. The client has a fever and chills after chemotherapy. What does the nurse give? Select all that apply.
    a. Aspirin
    b. Acetaminophen
    c. Demerol
    d. Erythropoietin
    e. Ibuprofen
    f. Naproxen

Answer: b. c. Acetaminophen can be given for fever and Demerol can be given for shaking chills. Aspirin and NSAIDs cannot be given because of the potential for thrombocytopenia.

Oncology Nursing

31. The client is having nausea from chemotherapy. What nursing interventions do you do?
    a. Tell the client to take antiemetics when vomiting.
    b. Instruct the client on relaxation techniques.
    c. Tell the client to lie down after eating.
    d. Tell the client to eat more sweet and spicy foods.

Answer: b. Instruct the client on relaxation techniques and take antiemetics around the clock. Sit up for thirty minutes after eating and eat fewer sweet, greasy, or spicy foods.

32. The client has stomatitis after chemotherapy. What can you tell the client?
    a. Use viscous xylocaine for pain relief.
    b. Eat plenty of popcorn and nuts.
    c. Suck on hard candy.
    d. Chew gum.

Answer: a. The client should use viscous xylocaine for pain relief. They should avoid popcorn, nuts, hard candy, and gum will only irritate the stomatitis.

33. The client is having constipation after chemotherapy. As the nurse, what do you suggest?
a. Avoid taking in fiber
b. Avoid dairy products
c. Take in extra dietary fiber
d. Restrict fluids

Answer: c. For constipation, take in extra fiber. Dairy products should be avoided in diarrhea. The client should drink extra fluids and take stool softeners.

34. The client is having problems coping because of her cancer diagnosis. How can the nurse help? Select all that apply.
a. Assess for suicide plans.
b. Assess for homicide plans.
c. Get a psychiatric and substance abuse history.
d. Encourage alcohol use in order to cope.
e. Monitor the client for evidence of depression.
f. Tell the client the symptoms will pass without intervention.

Answer: a. c. e. The client with coping problems may be depressed so you should look for evidence of depression and assess for suicide plans. Get a substance abuse history and encourage group support. Homicide is not usually a problem in cancer patients and alcohol can make things worse. Often, some kind of intervention is necessary.

35. A client is suffering from electrolyte complications of cancer. What is the most common electrolyte complication of cancer?
   a. Hypokalemia
   b. Hypocalcemia
   c. Hypernatremia
   d. Hypercalcemia

Answer: d. Up to 40 percent of all cancer patients will suffer from hypercalcemia. The others are not considered electrolyte complications of cancer.

36. The client is suffering from hypercalcemia from cancer. What does the nurse do about medications?
   a. Give bisphosphonates.
   b. Give extra digoxin.
   c. Avoid narcotic pain relief.
   d. Give medications with milk.

Answer: a. Bisphosphonates can decrease serum calcium levels. Clients are more sensitive to digoxin so you need to give less. Milk increases calcium levels and should be avoided. Narcotics can be given for pain.

37. The client with cancer has had mediastinal lymphadenopathy and has developed a sudden onset of shortness of breath, head swelling, swelling of the eyes, severe headache, neck, and arm swelling. What is most likely going on?
    a. Pulmonary embolism
    b. Pneumothorax
    c. Superior vena cava syndrome
    d. Rupture of the abdominal aorta

Answer: c. The client most likely has superior vena cava syndrome with a lack of blood return from the upper part of the body that normally is drained by the superior vena cava. The superior vena cava is most likely being impinged upon by mediastinal lymphadenopathy. The other choices do not carry the same constellation of symptoms.

38. The client has small cell cancer of the lung and has had a weight gain of greater than 5 pounds in one day, nausea and vomiting, confusion, fatigue, a serum sodium of 125 and decreased urinary output. What might be going on?
    a. Small cell cancer making inappropriate amounts of antidiuretic hormone (SIADH)
    b. Has been given too much IV fluids
    c. Kidney failure
    d. Kidney involvement in cancer

Answer: a. The client has SIADH from small cell cancer and is producing too much antidiuretic hormone. Too much IV fluids would give an increased urine output and renal failure or renal involvement in cancer would be much rarer in this type of cancer.

39. The client has SIADH from cancer. What are some nursing interventions that might be done?
   a. Increase IV fluids.
   b. Monitor blood for electrolyte imbalance.
   c. Give sugarless candy to better handle fluid restriction.
   d. Give hypotonic saline to bring down sodium level.
   e. Obtain daily weights.
   f. Give the client a high salt diet.

Answer: b. c. e. The client with SIADH needs fluid restriction and can be offered sugarless candy to cope with fluid restriction. Daily weights are indicated. The client does not need extra IV fluids nor do they need extra salt in spite of the fact that their sodium level will be low. Hypotonic saline would make the situation worse.

40. A client with leukemia has the acute onset of muscle twitching, seizures, lethargy, confusion and cardiac arrhythmias after receiving chemotherapy. What is going on?
   a. The client is having hypercalcemia from cancer.
   b. The client is suffering from tumor lysis syndrome.
   c. The client is getting too little fluid.
   d. The client is suffering from hypokalemia.

Answer: b. The client is suffering from tumor lysis syndrome, which can happen when tumor cells die and release large amounts of potassium, phosphorus, and uric acid into the bloodstream. This can result in cardiac arrhythmias from hyperkalemia and cardiac arrest. The potassium level will be high from tumor lysis. The calcium level will be low and this cannot be from dehydration.

41. The smoking client has gross hematuria that is painless and suprapubic, rectal and back pain. What do you suspect?
   a. Prostatitis
   b. UTI
   c. Transitional cell cancer of the bladder
   d. Pyelonephritis

Answer: c. The client needs a cystoscopy or urinary tumor cell evaluation for transitional cell cancer of the bladder. It is most often caused by smoking. Pyelonephritis would usually give flank pain and a UTI generally doesn't have painless hematuria. Prostatitis usually doesn't have gross hematuria.

42. The client has superficial transitional cell cancer of the bladder. What treatment would he likely get?
    a. Transurethral resection of the tumor and destruction of surrounding tumor.
    b. Radical cystectomy with removal of bladder, prostate, urethra, and seminal vesicles
    c. Brachytherapy
    d. BCG given intravesically for six weeks

Answer: d. For superficial transitional cell cancer of the bladder, BCG is often given intravesically for six weeks. The other treatments are for more advanced bladder cancer.

43. The male client is a smoker and has had excessive occupational exposure to lead cadmium and hematuria. What kind of cancer is he likely to have?
    a. Renal cell cancer
    b. Prostate cancer
    c. Bladder cancer
    d. Urethral cancer

Answer: a. Renal cell cancer is often found in men who have had occupational exposure to lead cadmium. His most likely early symptom is hematuria. Prostate, bladder, and urethral cancer are not found in patients with lead cadmium exposure and hematuria.

44. The client has metastatic renal cell cancer. What can you tell the client about sites of metastases?
   a. It usually spreads to the brain.
   b. It spreads by direct extension to the renal vein or vena cava.
   c. It usually spreads to the other kidney.
   d. It usually spreads via the blood to the bladder.

Answer: b. Renal cell cancer usually spreads by direct extension to the renal vein or vena cava. It does not commonly spread to the brain, the other kidney or to the bladder.

45. The female client has been diagnosed with breast cancer. What do you tell the client in order to educate her?
   a. It is the third most common cancer in women.
   b. Most cancers occur in the inner lower quadrant.
   c. Stage I and stage II disease are 70-90 percent curable.
   d. It is not capable of metastasis.

Answer: c. Stage I and stage II cancer of the breast are 70-90 percent curable. It is the most common cancer in women and it usually occurs in the upper outer quadrant of the breast. Advanced cases are capable of metastases.

46. The 75 year old female client has a red breast, with an orange-peel appearance to the skin and a painful breast. What could be going on?
    a. Ductal breast cancer
    b. Inflammatory breast cancer
    c. Lobular breast cancer
    d. Mastitis

Answer: b. Inflammatory breast cancer occurs in women who present with a red breast, an orange-peel appearance to the skin and a painful breast. Ductal and lobular breast cancer do not present this way and mastitis is rare in a 75 year old woman.

47. The client wants to know the most common areas of metastasis for her breast cancer? What do you say?
    a. Bone marrow, kidney, adrenal glands, gallbladder
    b. Bone, lung, liver, brain
    c. Brain only
    d. Intestines, pancreas, the other breast, gallbladder

Answer: b. The most common sites of metastasis for breast cancer are the bone, lung, liver and brain. The other sites are much less likely.

48. The client tells you she is scheduled for a simple mastectomy for her breast cancer and asks you what this means. What do you tell her?
    a. It involves the removal of the lump and some surrounding breast tissue.
    b. It involves the removal of the entire breast, including the nipple and the skin.
    c. It involves removal of the breast, the nipple, the skin and the axillary lymph nodes.
    d. It involves removal of the breast tissue, skin, lymph nodes and pectoral muscles.

Answer: b. A simple mastectomy involves removal of the breast, the nipple and the skin. A lumpectomy is removal of the lump and surrounding breast tissue only; a modified mastectomy includes the lymph nodes as well; a radical mastectomy includes removal of the pectoral muscles.

Oncology Nursing

49. The client with breast cancer is to have a sentinel lymph node biopsy. What do you tell her about this procedure?
    a. The largest lymph node in the axilla is removed to look for cancer.
    b. All the lymph nodes of the axilla are removed to look for cancer.
    c. Dye is injected in the lymph system, looking for the first draining axillary lymph node.
    d. Any lymph nodes that look suspicious for cancer are removed from the axilla.

Answer: c. In a sentinel lymph node biopsy, dye is injected into the lymph system, looking for the first draining axillary lymph node.

Oncology Nursing

50. The client is scheduled for radiation following lumpectomy. How do you educate the client abut this procedure?
    a. Tiny beads of radioactivity will be put beneath the skin at the time of surgery.
    b. Radiation is done during surgery to remove the breast.
    c. Radiation is done six months after the lump is removed if there is evidence of the cancer returning.
    d. External beam radiation is done about three weeks after the lump is removed.

Answer: d. If radiation is performed, it is done about three weeks after the lump is removed. This allows some time for surgical healing to take place.

51. The patient is being given Herceptin after treatment of breast cancer. How does the nurse explain the role of Herceptin?
    a. Tell her it is a form of chemotherapy for breast cancer.
    b. Tell her it is used to get rid of any cancer cells that weren't removed in surgery.
    c. Tell her it is a monoclonal antibody therapy used for tumors that express the HER2 oncogene.
    d. Tell her it is a hormone that blocks the growth of breast cancer cells.

Answer: c. Herceptin is a monoclonal antibody therapy that is used to stop the growth of tumors that express the HER2 gene.

52. The client recently underwent a CT scan for headaches that showed a mass on the brain. What do you tell the client about the brain mass?
    a. It is likely to be a malignant tumor.
    b. It is almost always fatal.
    c. Surgery will be used to remove the tumor.
    d. There are more metastatic brain cancers than primary brain cancers.

Answer: d. It is statistically more likely that the brain mass is a metastasis versus a primary brain cancer. Brain tumors can be benign or malignant and not all are fatal. Surgery and radiation are used to rid the brain of a brain tumor, regardless of cause.

53. The client has a metastatic brain tumor. He asks about the most common way of treating this type of condition. How do you respond?
   a. Most metastatic brain tumors are treated with radiation therapy.
   b. Most metastatic brain tumors are treated with chemotherapy.
   c. Most metastatic brain tumors are treated with stereotactic surgery.
   d. Most metastatic brain tumors are not treated at all.

Answer: a. Most metastatic treatments are treated with radiation therapy although some are resistant to radiation. Chemotherapy does not work on most brain cancers and stereotactic surgery is only done some of the time. The choice not to treat depends on the client.

54. The client with cervical cancer asks about her risk factors for the disease. What do you tell her about her risk factors? Select all that apply.
   a. Cigarette smoking is a risk factor.
   b. Human papillomavirus is a risk factor.
   c. Alcohol intake is a risk factor.
   d. High socioeconomic status is a risk factor
   e. Having multiple sex partners is a risk factor.
   f. Having sex after age 21 is a risk factor.

Answer: a. b. e. Risk factors for cervical cancer are cigarette smoking, human papillomavirus, low socioeconomic status, having multiple sexual partners and having sex before the age of 17.

55. The client is wondering about the best way to avoid getting cervical cancer. What do you say on prevention of cervical cancer?
   a. Avoid alcohol intake.
   b. Get a Pap smear upon becoming sexually active.
   c. Avoid douches.
   d. Get a routine colposcopy every 5 years.

Answer: b. The best prevention of cervical cancer is to have annual pap tests upon becoming sexually active. Colposcopy is done only if the Pap smear is abnormal. Avoiding douching and alcohol intake are not risk factors for cervical cancer.

56. The client is scheduled for a colposcopy. What do you tell the client in the way of education about colposcopy?
    a. Colposcopy is done under general anesthesia.
    b. Colposcopy involves putting a tube up the vagina and visualizing the cervix.
    c. Colposcopy involves putting acetic acid on the cervix and visualizing it under magnification.
    d. Colposcopy always results in removal of the cervix at the time of the procedure.

Answer: c. Colposcopy involves putting acetic acid on the cervix and visualizing it under magnification. It is done as an outpatient without general anesthesia. It can involve a biopsy but not removal of the entire cervix.

57. A 55 year old woman is diagnosed with cervical cancer. What is the main treatment of choice?
    a. Radiation to the pelvis.
    b. Removal of the cervix with sparing of the uterus.
    c. Cone biopsy of the cervix.
    d. Total abdominal hysterectomy and lymphadenectomy.

Answer: d. For a woman who is not of childbearing years, a total abdominal hysterectomy and lymphadenectomy is recommended. A cone biopsy is insufficient and radiation is not recommended.

Oncology Nursing

58. Nursing interventions for a client treated for cervical cancer include the following. Select all that apply?
    a. Measure all intake and output.
    b. Bladder retraining using a suprapubic catheter.
    c. Douche every 24 hours
    d. Assess for changes in bowel and bladder pattern after surgery/radiation.
    e. Avoid sex for 6 weeks.
    f. Teach how to use tampons after surgery.

Answer: b. d. Bladder retraining is necessary if the client has a suprapubic catheter. Intake and output does not have to be measured. No tampons, douching or sex for 2-4 weeks.

59. The client has been diagnosed with colon cancer and asks why he got the disease. What do you say in terms of risk factors for colon cancer?
    a. Eating a diet high in fish is a risk factor.
    b. Having a positive family history is a risk factor.
    c. Lupus is a risk factor.
    d. Eating lots of vegetables is a risk factor.

Answer: b. Having a diet high in red meat and low in vegetables is a risk factor for colon cancer as well as having Crohn's disease or ulcerative colitis. Lupus is not a risk factor. Having a family history of colon cancer is a risk factor for the disease.

60. The client has metastatic colon cancer. What is the most common site of metastatic colon cancer?
    a. Brain
    b. Pancreas
    c. Liver
    d. Lung

Answer: c. The most common site for metastatic colon cancer is the liver. Secondary sites include the bone, brain, and liver.

61. The client is asked about the best prevention of colon cancer. What do you tell the client?
    a. Drink no more than 2 alcoholic beverages per day.
    b. Have a FIT test every five years.
    c. Be seen if there is blood from the rectum.
    d. Have a colonoscopy every ten years after age 50.

Answer: The best prevention is to have a colonoscopy every ten years after age 50 to remove any precancerous polyps. Drinking less will reduce the risk factors. A FIT test is an alternative to a colonoscopy. By the time you have blood in the stool it may already mean you have colon cancer.

62. The client is having surgery to remove colon cancer the next day. What does the nurse expect to do?
    a. Give a Dulcolax suppository the night before the surgery.
    b. Give a GoLytely prep the day before the surgery.
    c. Give IV antibiotics on the day before the procedure.
    d. Restrict fluids the day before the procedure.

Answer: b. Oral antibiotics and a GoLytely prep should be given the day before surgery. A Dulcolax suppository is insufficient and IV antibiotics aren't given until the day of surgery. Fluids should be encouraged the day before surgery.

63. The client has colon cancer in the sigmoid colon. What procedure is the client likely to have to treat this condition?
    a. Left hemicolectomy
    b. Sigmoidectomy
    c. Right hemicolectomy
    d. Total colectomy

Answer: a. The treatment of left-sided colon cancer is always a left hemicolectomy. Sigmoidectomy is not enough an a total colectomy is too much. The right hemicolectomy is on the wrong side of the affected colon.

Oncology Nursing

64. Priority nursing interventions for a client who is undergoing colon surgery for colon cancer includes:
    a. Tell them to expect normal sexual function after recovery.
    b. Watch for an anastomotic leak from the site of the surgical re-connect.
    c. Educate the client on eating after surgery.
    d. Monitor for bladder dysfunction.

Answer: b. After surgery, monitor the client for anastomotic leak (fever, abdominal pain). Expect some sexual dysfunction. Education on diet is not a priority right after surgery. Bladder dysfunction is not expected.

65. The client is at risk for endometrial cancer. What are her risks?
    a. Being younger than age 30.
    b. Having multiple children.
    c. Being African-American.
    d. Having a family history of breast or ovarian cancer.

Answer: d. There are several risk factors for endometrial cancer, including being Caucasian, being older than age 50, being infertile, being nulliparous, having obesity, diabetes, and hypertension.

66. Common metastatic sites for endometrial cancer include the following:
    a. Cervix and vagina
    b. Colon
    c. Liver
    d. Brain

Answer: a. The most common sites of metastases from endometrial cancer includes the cervix and the vagina.

67. The best method of detecting endometrial cancer is what?
    a. A Pap smear
    b. An endometrial biopsy
    c. A hysterectomy
    d. Vaginal washings

Answer: b. An endometrial biopsy detects endometrial cancer 90 percent of the time and is the best method of detecting endometrial cancer. Hysterectomy is a treatment for the disease.

68. The client has gastric cancer and wonders about his risks for getting the disease. What are they?
   a. Female gender
   b. Being Caucasian
   c. Having a Helicobacter infection
   d. Having colon cancer

Answer: c. Risk factors for the disease include being African-American, Japanese, Chinese, Hawaiian, male over the age of 40, poor nutritional habits, family history, previous gastric resection, pernicious anemia, gastric atrophy, gastritis, and a Helicobacter pylori. Being a rubber worker or coal miner are risk factors as well.

69. The client has metastatic gastric cancer. Where is a likely metastasis?
   a. Pancreas
   b. Bone
   c. Brain
   d. Lung

Answer: a. Pancreas, esophagus, and liver are the main sites of metastases from gastric cancer because it spreads through direct extension.

Oncology Nursing

70. The client has cancer of the larynx and wonders how he got it. What is a main risk factor for laryngeal cancer?
    a. Eating a low fiber diet
    b. Having laryngeal polyps
    c. Smoking history
    d. Illicit drug use

Answer: c. Smoking and drinking account for 95 percent of these types of cancers.

71. The client has metastatic cancer of the larynx. Where is the major site of metastasis?
    a. Bone
    b. Brain
    c. Other head and neck areas
    d. Colon

Answer: c. The most likely metastasis of laryngeal cancer is local spread to other head and neck areas. Distant metastatic spread is rare.

72. The client has persistent hoarseness, throat pain, and a painless mass in the neck. What is the most likely diagnosis?
    a. Laryngeal polyp
    b. Laryngeal cancer
    c. Tonsillitis
    d. Esophagitis

Answer: b. Persistent hoarseness, throat pain, and a painless mass, especially in the presence of tobacco and alcohol use is high risk for laryngeal cancer.

73. The client has nasopharyngeal cancer. What can he expect as the main form of therapy?
    a. Removal of the voice box.
    b. Radiation to the head and neck.
    c. Interleukin-2
    d. Cisplatin

Answer: b. All are treatments for nasopharyngeal cancer but radiation treatment is considered the primary treatment.

74. The client has weight loss, unexplained bleeding, splenomegaly, anemia, low platelet count and a WBC count of 50,000. What do you expect is going on?
    a. Hodgkin's lymphoma
    b. Anorexia nervosa
    c. Non-Hodgkin's lymphoma
    d. Acute leukemia

Answer: d. The symptoms of weight loss, unexplained bleeding, anemia, low platelet count and high WBC count are most consistent with acute leukemia.

75. The primary treatment for leukemia and multiple myeloma is what?
    a. Lymph node surgery
    b. Chemotherapy alone
    c. Chemotherapy and radiation
    d. Chemotherapy and bone marrow transplant

Answer: d. The primary treatment for leukemia and multiple myeloma is chemotherapy followed by bone marrow transplant.

Oncology Nursing

76. The client has been diagnosed with lung cancer and wonders how he got it. What does the nurse say about the primary cause of lung cancer?
    a. Cigarette smoking
    b. Radon gas
    c. Asbestos exposure
    d. Secondhand smoke

Answer: a. Cigarette smoking is the number one cause of lung cancer, while the other causes are secondary factors.

77. The client is suspected of having lung cancer by a suspicious x-ray of the chest. What follow up test is most appropriate to detect whether or not the suspicious area is cancer?
    a. Repeat CXR in six months.
    b. Bronchoscopy with biopsy.
    c. Sputum culture.
    d. Lobectomy of the lung.

Answer: b. A bronchoscopy with biopsy is a good follow up test to identify cancer in a suspicious lesion.

78. The client has been diagnosed with localized small cell cancer. What is the standard treatment for this disease?
   a. Pneumonectomy
   b. Lobectomy
   c. Chemotherapy
   d. Brachytherapy

Answer: c. Chemotherapy is the standard treatment for small cell cancer. Surgery and brachytherapy are not recommended but radiation can be used in small cell cancer as well.

79. Nursing interventions for those who have had a lobectomy for lung cancer include the following:
   a. Lie on the side of the operation for better drainage.
   b. Encourage a reduction in smoking.
   c. Manage chest tubes in lobectomy.
   d. Keep the client in bed for at least a week.

Answer: c. In a lobectomy, the client should lie on the opposite side of the surgery and should encourage the stoppage of smoking altogether. Breathing, coughing and ambulation are important as is managing the chest tubes.

80. The client has been diagnosed with ovarian cancer. How do you educate the client about the disease?
   a. The peak age is 80-89 years of age.
   b. A total of 60-70 percent of people are diagnosed at stage III or IV.
   c. Being multiparous is a risk factor.
   d. The five year survival rate is 80 percent.

Answer: b. A total of 60-70 percent of people are diagnosed at stage III or IV. The peak age at onset is 55-59. There are no risk factors. The five year survival rate is 30-35 percent.

81. The client has metastatic cervical cancer. Where are the most likely site(s) for metastasis of this type of cancer?
   a. Extension to fallopian tubes, uterus, bladder and peritoneum
   b. Bone
   c. Brain
   d. Liver

Answer: a. The most likely site of cancer metastasis of cervical cancer is fallopian tubes, uterus, bladder, and peritoneum.

82. The routine treatment for ovarian cancer is what?
    a. Brachytherapy at the site of cancer
    b. Radiation to the abdomen
    c. Total abdominal hysterectomy and bilateral oophorectomy
    d. Chemotherapy in the peritoneum

Answer: c. The main therapy for ovarian cancer is a total abdominal hysterectomy and bilateral oophorectomy.

83. The client has discovered he has prostate cancer and wants to know details. How do you educate him on the disease?
    a. It has the highest rate in Caucasians.
    b. It has a nearly 100 percent 5 year survival rate.
    c. It is the leading cause of cancer death in men.
    d. It is most common in men under the age of 65.

Answer: b. Prostate cancer has a nearly 100 percent survival rate but is still the second leading cause of cancer death. It is much more common in African-Americans. It is most common in men older than 65.

84. The client has metastatic prostate cancer. What is the major site of prostate cancer metastases?
    a. Bone
    b. Brain
    c. Pancreas
    d. Omentum

Answer: a. A large amount of prostate cancer patients have metastases to bones. It can go to the liver, lung, and bladder as well.

85. The client has a weak urinary stream and an inability to start or stop the flow of urine. He has frequent nocturia and hematuria. What kind of cancer might he have?
    a. Bladder cancer
    b. Kidney cancer
    c. Urethral cancer
    d. Prostate cancer

Answer: d. The symptoms are most consistent with prostate cancer.

86. Surgical management of prostate cancer include what?
   a. Radical prostatectomy
   b. Lymph node removal of the pelvic lymph nodes
   c. Transurethral resection of the prostate
   d. Only radiation surgery is recommended

Answer: a. The main surgical management of prostate cancer involves a radical prostatectomy, which removes the prostate, the seminal vesicles, some lymph nodes, and ejaculatory ducts.

87. Adjuvant therapy for prostate cancer includes:
   a. Removal of urethra.
   b. External beam radiation of the bladder
   c. Hormonal manipulation
   d. Removal of the bladder

Answer: c. Adjuvant therapy for prostate cancer includes brachytherapy and hormonal therapy, which can involve giving estrogen and removing the testes. Leuprolide and goserelin can be given as part of hormonal manipulation of prostate cancer.

Oncology Nursing

88. Nursing interventions for prostate cancer clients include the following:
    a. Teach the client how to remove the catheter after surgery.
    b. Keep client in bed for 48 hours after surgery.
    c. Give laxatives for constipation.
    d. Report to physician if client has evidence of infection after brachytherapy.

Answer: d. The client is to have a urinary catheter for several weeks after surgery. The client should ambulate as soon as possible after surgery and should turn and cough regularly. Laxatives should not be given but stool softeners are acceptable. Report to physician voiding difficulties and evidence of infection after receiving brachytherapy.

89. After brachytherapy for prostate cancer, the client should be instructed by telling him this:
    a. The brachytherapy seeds pose a hazard to those around him.
    b. The client can be around pregnant women after receiving brachytherapy.
    c. Strain the urine for dislodged seeds.
    d. The client can be discharged immediately after receiving brachytherapy.

Answer: c. The client should be kept in the hospital until radioactivity decreases. The client is not a radioactive hazard to those around him but should stay away from pregnant women and children as a precaution. Strain the urine and wear a condom to look for dislodged seeds.

Oncology Nursing

90. The client has been diagnosed with skin cancer. How do you educate the client as to skin cancer?
    a. Melanoma is the most common type of skin cancer.
    b. Basal cell carcinoma is often fatal.
    c. Seborrheic keratoses can lead to squamous cell cancer.
    d. Actinic keratoses can lead to squamous cell cancer.

Answer: d. Actinic keratoses can lead to squamous cell cancer. Seborrheic keratoses do not lead to cancer. Basal cell cancer is practically never fatal. Melanoma is the third most common skin cancer.

91. The client has been diagnosed with melanoma. How do you educate the client on melanoma?
    a. The rate is highest among African-Americans.
    b. The melanoma arises from cells in the epidermis.
    c. It is more common in women than men.
    d. It cannot be prevented.

Answer: c. Melanoma is most common among women who are Caucasian. It arises from melanocytes in the dermis of the skin. It can be prevented by wearing hats and using sunscreen.

92. Risk factors for melanoma include:
    a. Wearing sunscreen in adulthood only.
    b. Getting bad sunburns in childhood.
    c. Having a darker complexion
    d. Getting sunburn in older age.

Answer: b. Risk factors for melanoma include excessive exposure to UVA and UVB rays, not wearing sunscreen, getting bad sunburns in childhood, having a fair complexion, having HIV, and being exposed in the workplace to various chemicals. Having atypical nevi is also a risk factor.

93. Melanoma can be identified by what characteristics?
    a. Non-uniform color of lesions
    b. Symmetric expansion of a mole
    c. Regular borders in the mole.
    d. Pearly appearance to the nodule.

Answer: a. Melanoma lesions have irregular, asymmetric borders and a non-uniform color to the lesion. Pearly lesions are common in basal cell carcinoma.

94. Treatment of a basal cell or squamous cell skin cancer includes:
    a. Radiation only
    b. Punch biopsy to the lesion.
    c. Wide excision to include healthy tissue
    d. Chemotherapy only

Answer: c. The treatment of a basal cell or squamous cell cancer involves making a wide excision to include healthy tissue. A punch biopsy is insufficient and chemotherapy/radiation are rarely used.

95. Common adjuvant therapy for melanoma cancer includes:
    a. External beam radiation
    b. Brachytherapy
    c. Chemotherapy
    d. Removal of lymph nodes

Answer: a. External beam radiation is a commonly used form of adjuvant therapy for melanoma. Brachytherapy is not used. Chemotherapy often fails and removal of lymph nodes is part of primary therapy and staging for melanoma.

96. The patient has been diagnosed with osteosarcoma. Where is the tumor originating from?
    a. Cartilage
    b. Bone
    c. Fibrous tissue
    d. Reticuloendothelial tissue

Answer: b. Osteosarcoma originates in bone. Chondrosarcoma originates in cartilage. Fibrosarcoma originates in fibrous tissue, and Ewing's sarcoma originates in reticuloendothelial tissue.

97. The client has been diagnosed with osteosarcoma. How do you educate the client with regard to this tumor?
    a. It is a common form of cancer.
    b. It is the most common bone tumor.
    c. The survival rate is 25 percent after five years.
    d. It does not require chemotherapy.

Answer: b. Osteosarcoma is rare but is the most common bone tumor. The survival rate with chemotherapy is 50 percent. Chemotherapy is used to treat the cancer.

98. The client has osteosarcoma and wonders about risk factors for the disease. What do you say?
    a. It is most common after the age of 50.
    b. It is most common in females.
    c. Previous radiation is a risk factor.
    d. Older adults never get the disease.

Answer: c. The disease is most common in males between the ages of 10 and 25 and in older adults who have Paget's disease. Previous radiation is a risk factor.

99. The client has metastatic osteosarcoma. What do you say about the most common metastatic sites?
    a. It is mostly metastatic to lungs.
    b. It is most metastatic to brain.
    c. It is most metastatic to liver.
    d. It is most metastatic to bowel tissue.

Answer: a. Osteosarcoma is usually metastatic to the lungs. It is rarely metastatic to bowel, liver, or brain.

Oncology Nursing

100. Nursing interventions for soft tissue sarcomas include what? Select all that apply.
   a. Emotional support for changes in body image.
   b. Increase fluids after surgery.
   c. Collaborate with speech therapy.
   d. Teach transfer techniques after surgery.
   e. Prepare the client for phantom limb pain if amputation is done.
   f. Monitor electrolytes.

Answer: a. d. e. The nurse should provide emotional support for changes in body image and should collaborate with occupational and physical therapy. Teach transfer techniques after surgery and prepare the client for phantom limb pain after surgery if amputation is done. Fluid increase and electrolyte monitoring are not exclusive to sarcomas and speech therapy is generally not required.

Oncology Nursing

101. The client has been diagnosed with testicular cancer. How do you educate the client about this type of cancer?
    a. It is a common male cancer.
    b. It occurs most often in men between the ages of 15 and 35.
    c. It is a non-aggressive tumor.
    d. It has the highest incidence in African-Americans.

Answer: b. Testicular cancer is most often occurring in Caucasian men between the ages of 15 and 35. The incidence is highest in Scandinavian countries. The cancer is rare but is very aggressive. It is curable if caught early.

102. The male client has found a small, hard scrotal mass. What do you suspect?
    a. Varicocele
    b. Testicular cancer
    c. Undescended testicle
    d. Testicular torsion

Answer: b. A small hard, scrotal mass is most consistent with testicular cancer. An undescended testicle is a risk factor for testicular cancer. A varicocele is not hard to the touch and testicular torsion is pain and swelling of the entire testicle.

Oncology Nursing

103. A common blood test for testicular cancer is what?
    a. Serum alkaline phosphatase
    b. Serum CA-125
    c. Serum LDH level
    d. Serum beta HCG

Answer: d. Blood tests for serum alpha fetoprotein or beta HCG are elevated in 85 percent of cases of testicular cancer.

104. The client asks the nurse about mortality from cancer. How does the nurse respond?
    a. About 5 million people in the US survive cancer for five years or more.
    b. Everyone in the US with cancer will eventually die from their disease.
    c. Cancer is the leading cause of adult death in the US.
    d. Do not discuss mortality with clients who have cancer.

Answer: a. About five million people diagnosed with cancer each year will live for five years or more.

105. The client indicates that he has heard that all men get prostate cancer at some point in their lives. How does the nurse educate the client?
   a. Lung cancer is the most frequently diagnosed cancer in men.
   b. Prostate cancer is the most frequently diagnosed cancer in men.
   c. Prostate cancer is most common in Caucasian men.
   d. As there is no way to screen for prostate cancer, it is the number one cause of cancer death in men.

Answer: b. Prostate cancer is the most frequently diagnosed cancer in men. Lung cancer is second. It is more common among African-Americans and there is screening available for this cancer.

Conclusion

I hope you received a ton of value from this book. Remember, practice makes perfect so you will have to repeat these readings.

If you enjoyed this book, would you be kind enough to leave a review on Amazon? Your positive review can help others to see what kinds of helpful resources are out there!

Thank you and good luck on your medical endeavors!

- Chase Hassen

Nurse Superhero

Oncology Nursing

Highly Recommended Books for Success

1. NCLEX: Cardiovascular System : 105 Nursing Practice and Rationales to Easily Crush the NCLEX!

2. NCLEX: Emergency Nursing : 105 Practice Questions and Rationales to Easily Crush the NCLEX!

3. Lab Values: 137 Values You Know to Easily Pass The NCLEX!

4. EKG Interpretation: 24 Hours or Less to Easily Pass the ECG Portion of the NCLEX!

5. Fluid and Electrolytes: 24 Hours or Less to Absolutely Crush the NCLEX Exam!

6. Nursing Careers: Easily Choose What Nursing Career Will Make Your 12 Hour Shift a Blast!

7. Night Shift: 10 Survival Tips for Nurses to Get Through The Night!

8. NCLEX: Endocrine System : 105 Nursing Practice Questions and Rationales to EASILY Crush the NCLEX!

And **MUCH MUCH MORE**! Visit my amazon author page to see more at http://amzn.to/1HCtfSy

Made in the USA
Las Vegas, NV
26 March 2022